Log it

FITNESS LOG BOOK

FIRST PUBLISHED 2020

DESIGNED BY GEORGINA BARNES

ILLUSTRATIONS ON COVER PAGE ©ANNA VALENTY,
KETTLEBELL ILLUSTRATION ON BODY CHECK,
PB CHCKER AND WORKOUT PAGES ©ICONICBESTIARY
& BODY ILLUSTRATION ©IRINA MIR.

ISBN: 978-1-71658-554-8

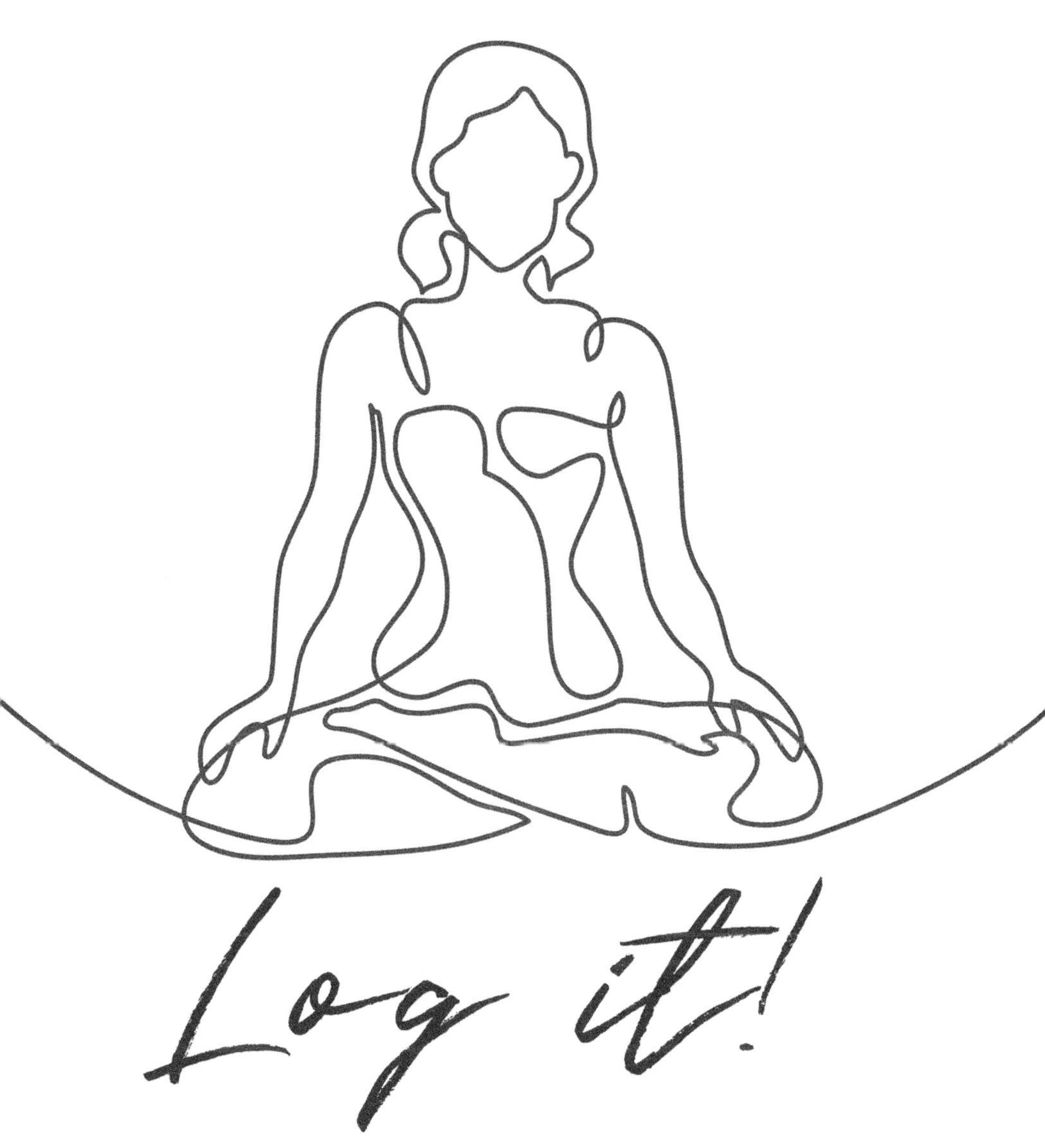

Log it!

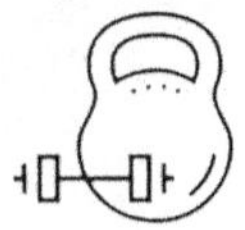

BODY CHECK

"Loving yourself is the greatest revolution."

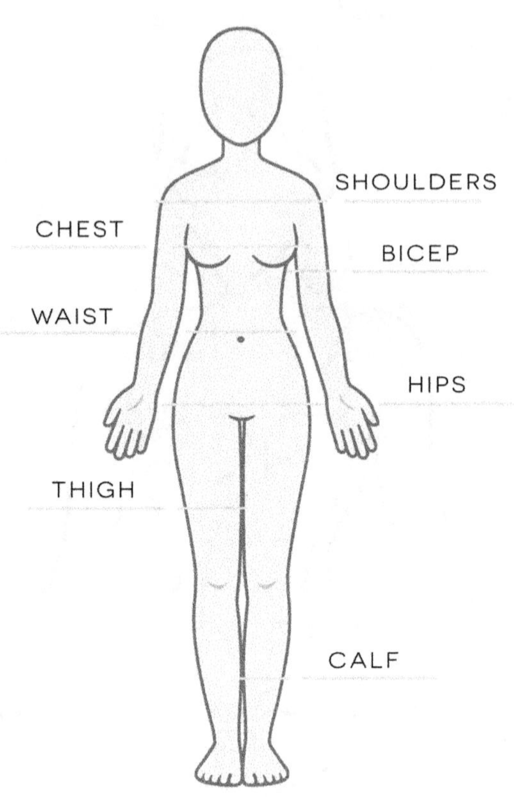

SHOULDERS									
CHEST									
BICEP									
WAIST									
HIPS									
THIGH									
CALF									

Notes

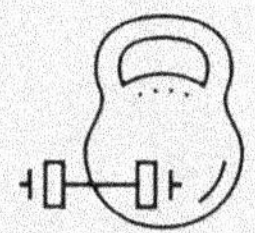

WORK

ON YOU

FOR

you.

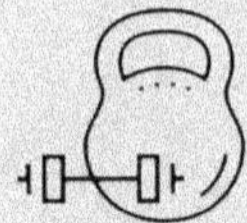

THE GREATEST WEALTH IS *Health.*

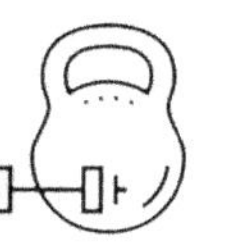

PR TRACKER

"Strength is beautiful."

EXERCISE

Notes

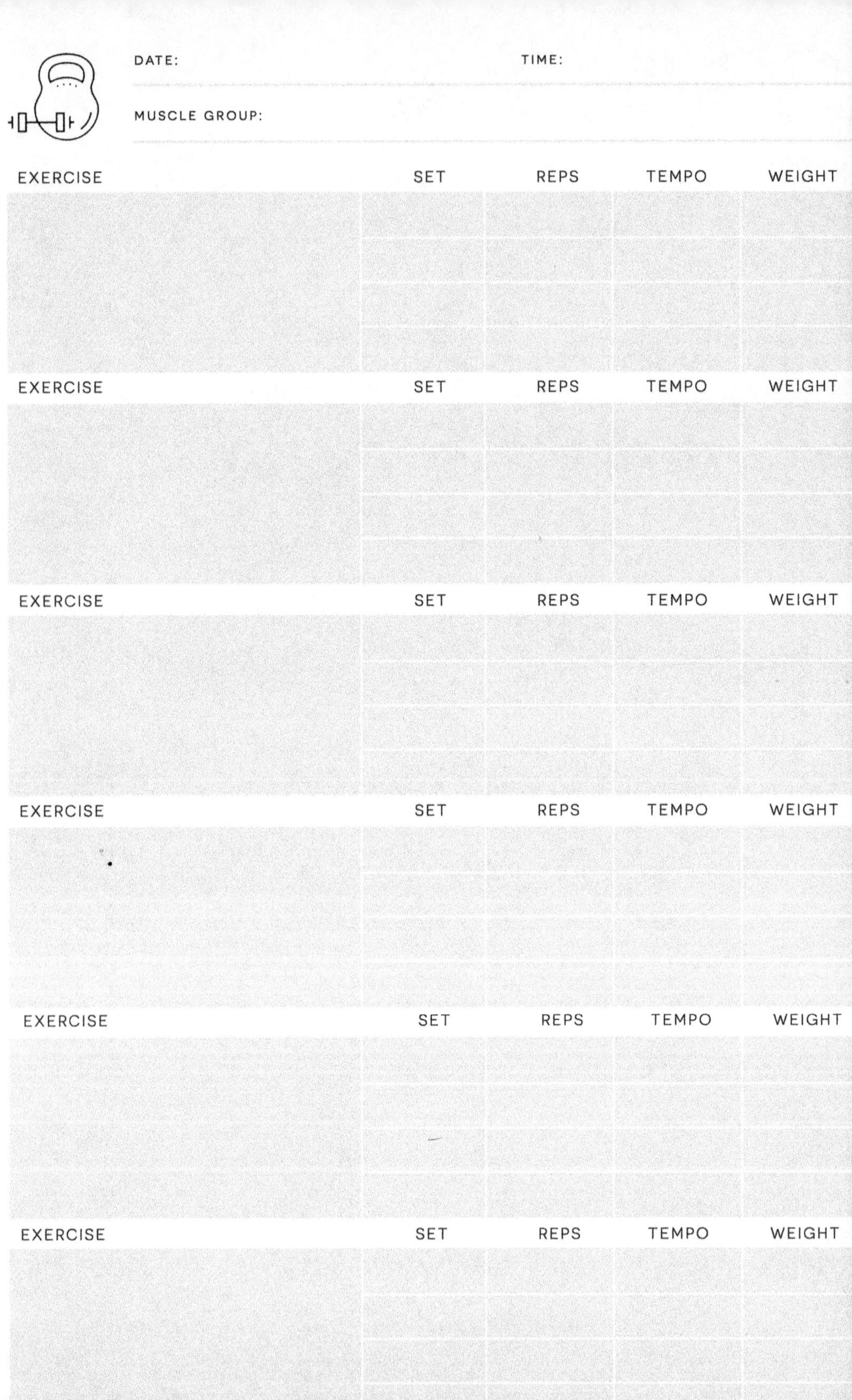

DATE:
TIME:
MUSCLE GROUP:

EXERCISE | SET | REPS | TEMPO | WEIGHT

EXERCISE | SET | REPS | TEMPO | WEIGHT

EXERCISE | SET | REPS | TEMPO | WEIGHT

EXERCISE | SET | REPS | TEMPO | WEIGHT

EXERCISE | SET | REPS | TEMPO | WEIGHT

EXERCISE | SET | REPS | TEMPO | WEIGHT

"Dear Body, 1 love you!

EXERCISE	SET	REPS	TEMPO	WEIGHT

EXERCISE	SET	REPS	TEMPO	WEIGHT

EXERCISE	SET	REPS	TEMPO	WEIGHT

EXERCISE	SET	REPS	TEMPO	WEIGHT

Notes

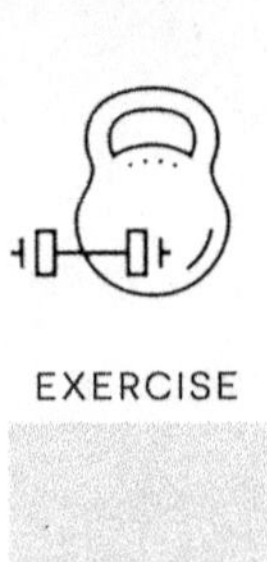

EXERCISE		SET	REPS	TEMPO	WEIGHT

EXERCISE		SET	REPS	TEMPO	WEIGHT

EXERCISE		SET	REPS	TEMPO	WEIGHT

EXERCISE		SET	REPS	TEMPO	WEIGHT

EXERCISE		SET	REPS	TEMPO	WEIGHT

EXERCISE		SET	REPS	TEMPO	WEIGHT

"Dear Body, I love you!"

EXERCISE		SET	REPS	TEMPO	WEIGHT

EXERCISE		SET	REPS	TEMPO	WEIGHT

EXERCISE		SET	REPS	TEMPO	WEIGHT

EXERCISE		SET	REPS	TEMPO	WEIGHT

Notes

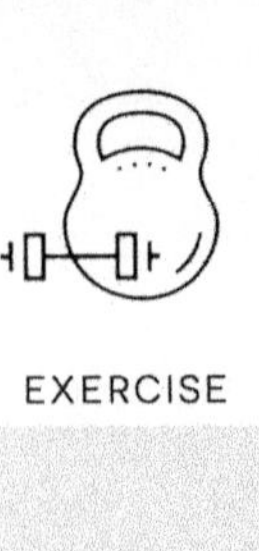

DATE:

TIME:

MUSCLE GROUP:

EXERCISE	SET	REPS	TEMPO	WEIGHT

EXERCISE	SET	REPS	TEMPO	WEIGHT

EXERCISE	SET	REPS	TEMPO	WEIGHT

EXERCISE	SET	REPS	TEMPO	WEIGHT

EXERCISE	SET	REPS	TEMPO	WEIGHT

EXERCISE	SET	REPS	TEMPO	WEIGHT

"Dear Body, I love you!"

EXERCISE	SET	REPS	TEMPO	WEIGHT

EXERCISE	SET	REPS	TEMPO	WEIGHT

EXERCISE	SET	REPS	TEMPO	WEIGHT

EXERCISE	SET	REPS	TEMPO	WEIGHT

Notes

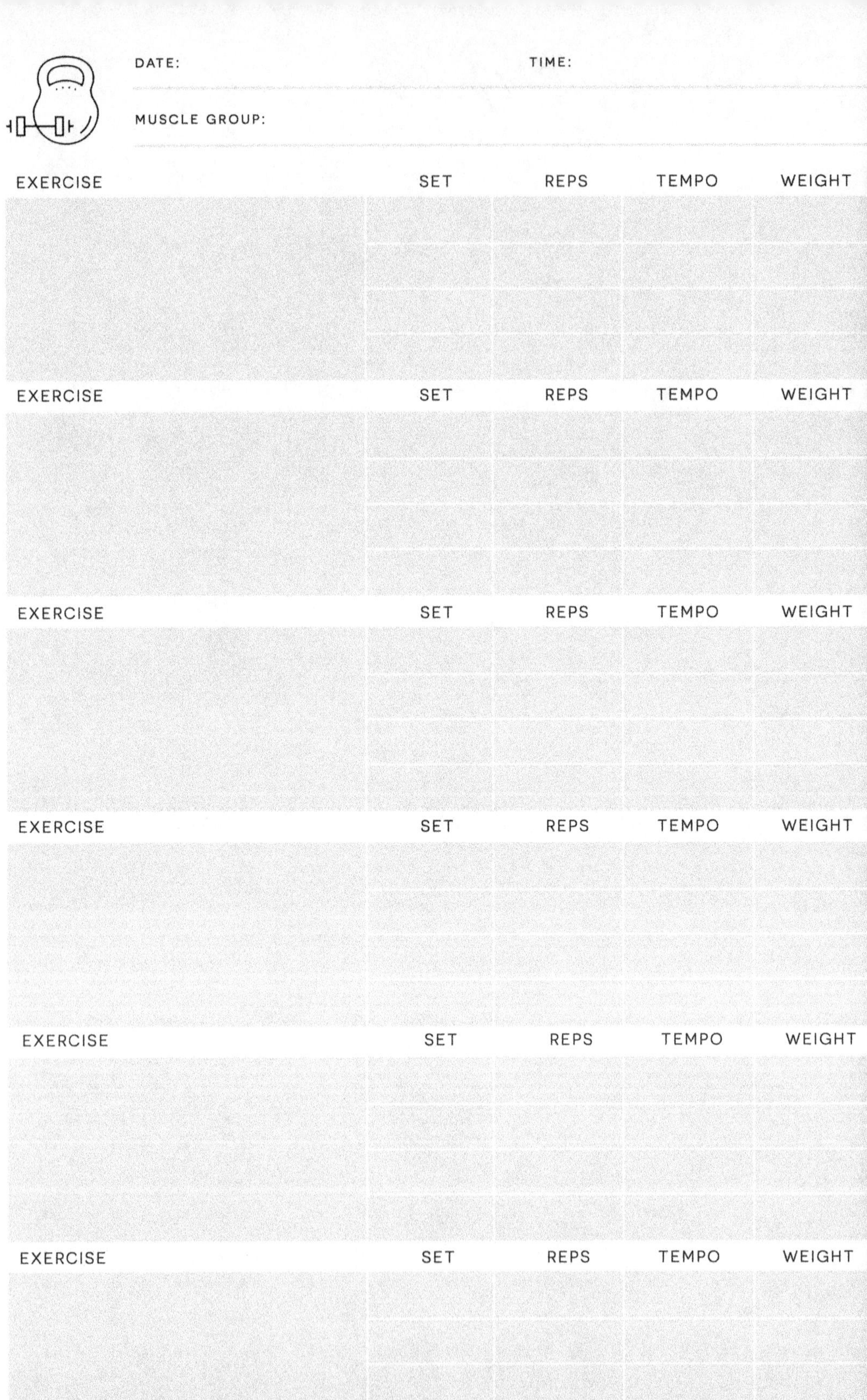

DATE:
TIME:
MUSCLE GROUP:

EXERCISE
SET
REPS
TEMPO
WEIGHT

EXERCISE
SET
REPS
TEMPO
WEIGHT

EXERCISE
SET
REPS
TEMPO
WEIGHT

EXERCISE
SET
REPS
TEMPO
WEIGHT

EXERCISE
SET
REPS
TEMPO
WEIGHT

EXERCISE
SET
REPS
TEMPO
WEIGHT

EXERCISE	SET	REPS	TEMPO	WEIGHT

EXERCISE	SET	REPS	TEMPO	WEIGHT

EXERCISE	SET	REPS	TEMPO	WEIGHT

EXERCISE	SET	REPS	TEMPO	WEIGHT

Notes

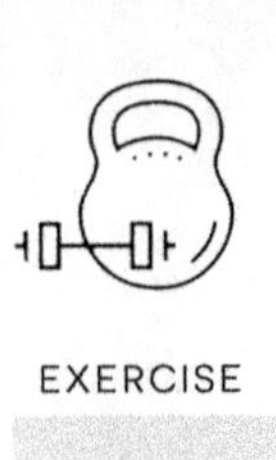

EXERCISE	SET	REPS	TEMPO	WEIGHT

EXERCISE	SET	REPS	TEMPO	WEIGHT

EXERCISE	SET	REPS	TEMPO	WEIGHT

EXERCISE	SET	REPS	TEMPO	WEIGHT

EXERCISE	SET	REPS	TEMPO	WEIGHT

EXERCISE	SET	REPS	TEMPO	WEIGHT

EXERCISE	SET	REPS	TEMPO	WEIGHT

EXERCISE	SET	REPS	TEMPO	WEIGHT

EXERCISE	SET	REPS	TEMPO	WEIGHT

EXERCISE	SET	REPS	TEMPO	WEIGHT

Notes

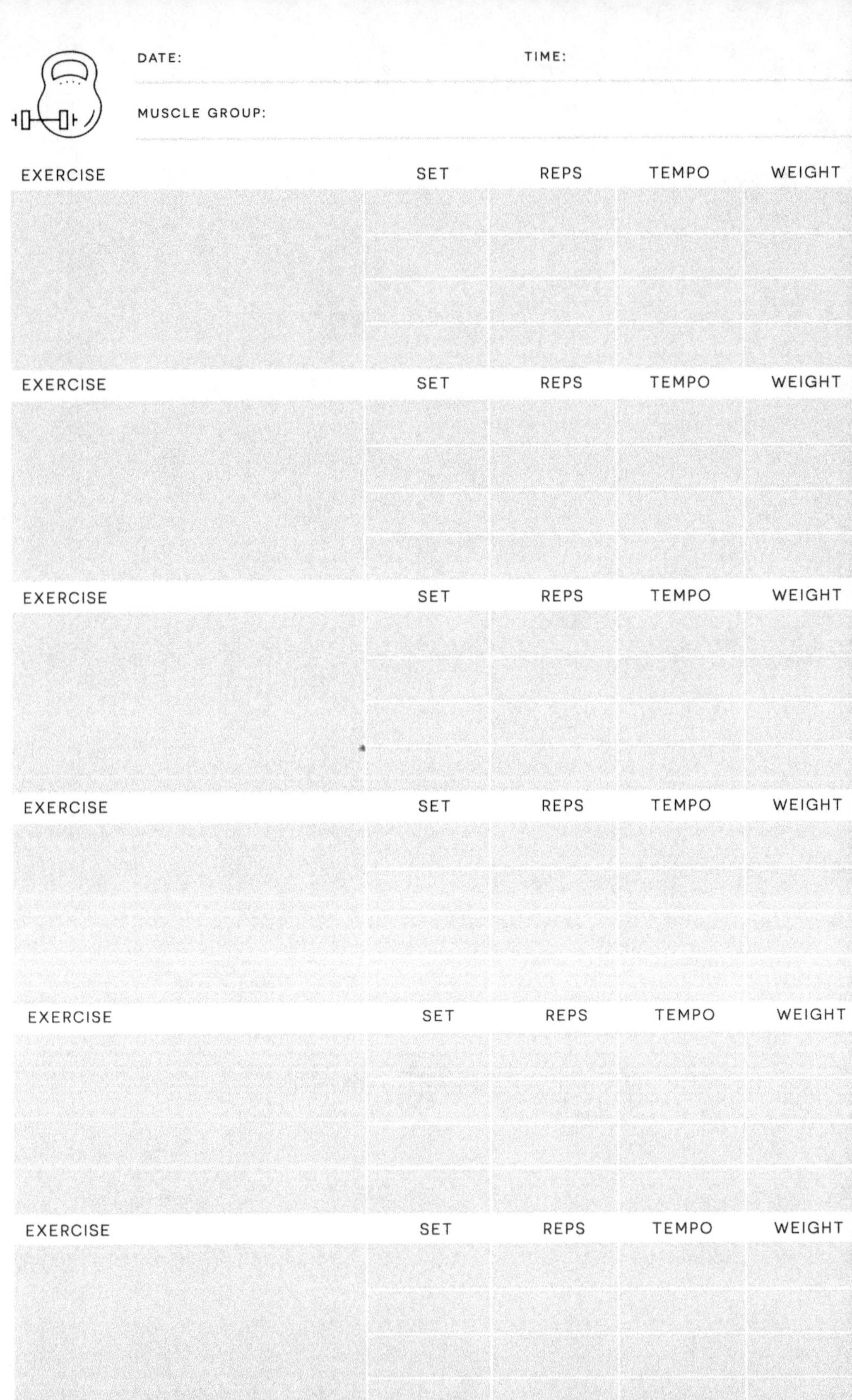

DATE:
TIME:
MUSCLE GROUP:
EXERCISE
SET
REPS
TEMPO
WEIGHT
EXERCISE
SET
REPS
TEMPO
WEIGHT
EXERCISE
SET
REPS
TEMPO
WEIGHT
EXERCISE
SET
REPS
TEMPO
WEIGHT
EXERCISE
SET
REPS
TEMPO
WEIGHT
EXERCISE
SET
REPS
TEMPO
WEIGHT

"Dear Body, I love you!"

EXERCISE	SET	REPS	TEMPO	WEIGHT

EXERCISE	SET	REPS	TEMPO	WEIGHT

EXERCISE	SET	REPS	TEMPO	WEIGHT

EXERCISE	SET	REPS	TEMPO	WEIGHT

Notes

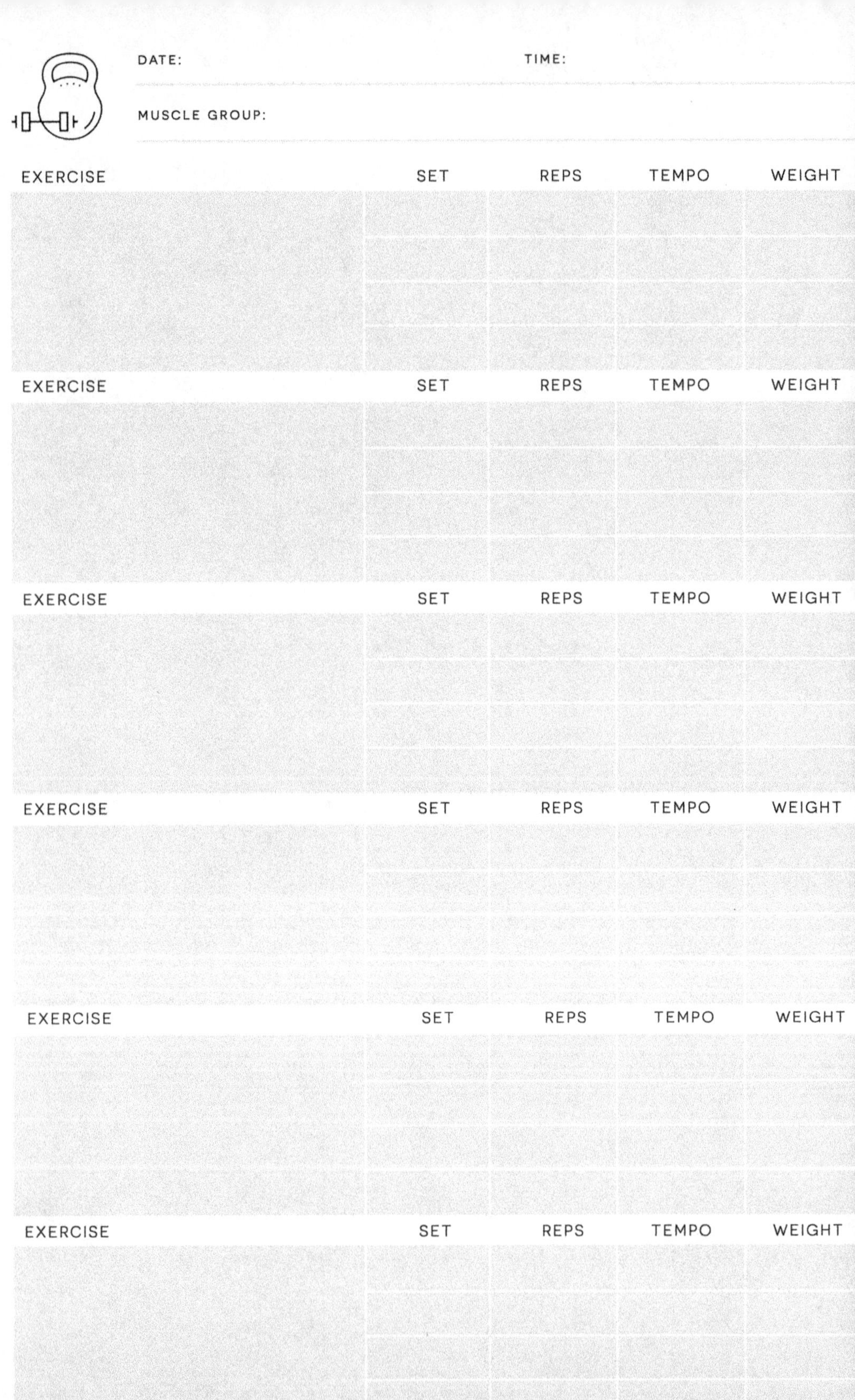

EXERCISE	SET	REPS	TEMPO	WEIGHT

EXERCISE	SET	REPS	TEMPO	WEIGHT

EXERCISE	SET	REPS	TEMPO	WEIGHT

EXERCISE	SET	REPS	TEMPO	WEIGHT

EXERCISE	SET	REPS	TEMPO	WEIGHT

EXERCISE	SET	REPS	TEMPO	WEIGHT

"Dear Body, I love you!"

EXERCISE		SET	REPS	TEMPO	WEIGHT

EXERCISE		SET	REPS	TEMPO	WEIGHT

EXERCISE		SET	REPS	TEMPO	WEIGHT

EXERCISE		SET	REPS	TEMPO	WEIGHT

Notes

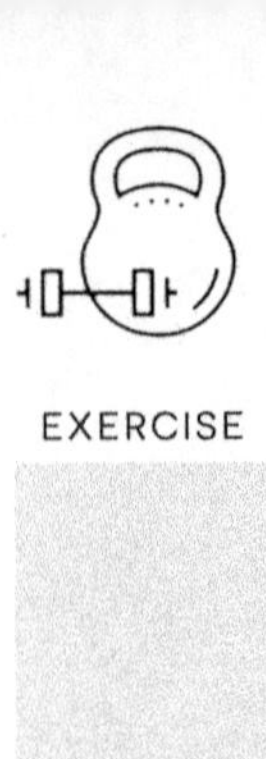

EXERCISE	SET	REPS	TEMPO	WEIGHT

EXERCISE	SET	REPS	TEMPO	WEIGHT

EXERCISE	SET	REPS	TEMPO	WEIGHT

EXERCISE	SET	REPS	TEMPO	WEIGHT

EXERCISE	SET	REPS	TEMPO	WEIGHT

EXERCISE	SET	REPS	TEMPO	WEIGHT

"Dear Body, I love you!"

EXERCISE	SET	REPS	TEMPO	WEIGHT

EXERCISE	SET	REPS	TEMPO	WEIGHT

EXERCISE	SET	REPS	TEMPO	WEIGHT

EXERCISE	SET	REPS	TEMPO	WEIGHT

Notes

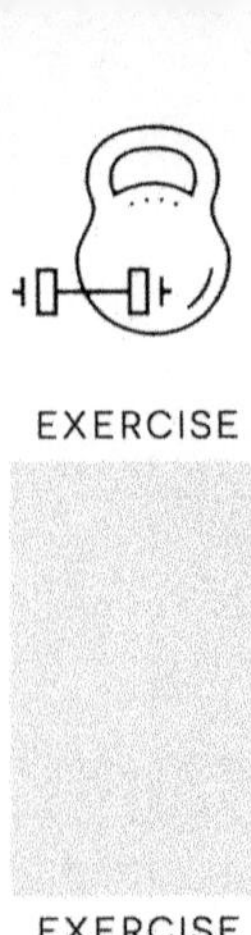

DATE: TIME:

MUSCLE GROUP:

EXERCISE	SET	REPS	TEMPO	WEIGHT

EXERCISE	SET	REPS	TEMPO	WEIGHT

EXERCISE	SET	REPS	TEMPO	WEIGHT

EXERCISE	SET	REPS	TEMPO	WEIGHT

EXERCISE	SET	REPS	TEMPO	WEIGHT

EXERCISE	SET	REPS	TEMPO	WEIGHT

"Dear Body, I love you!"

EXERCISE	SET	REPS	TEMPO	WEIGHT

EXERCISE	SET	REPS	TEMPO	WEIGHT

EXERCISE	SET	REPS	TEMPO	WEIGHT

EXERCISE	SET	REPS	TEMPO	WEIGHT

Notes

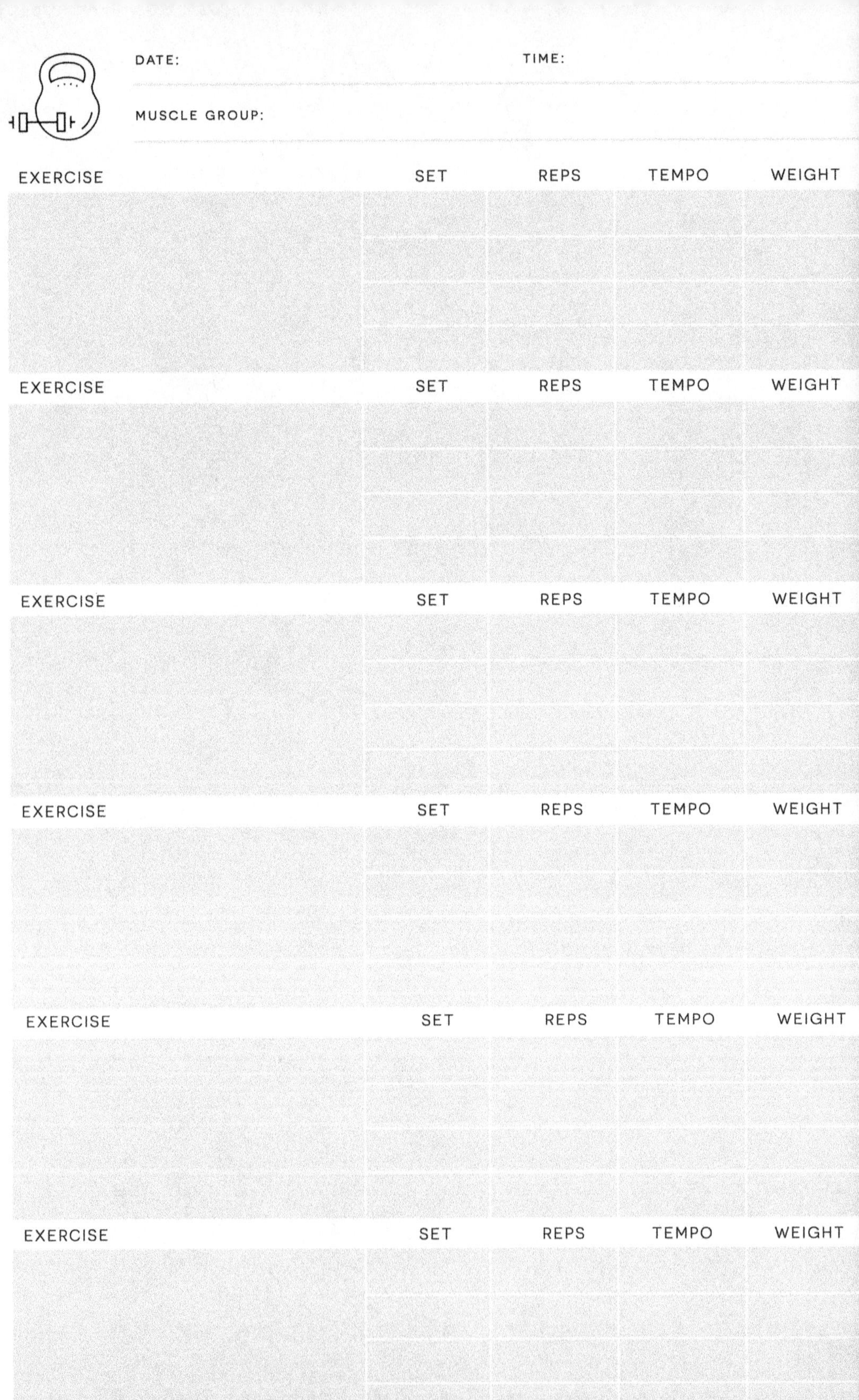

DATE:
TIME:
MUSCLE GROUP:

EXERCISE   SET   REPS   TEMPO   WEIGHT

EXERCISE   SET   REPS   TEMPO   WEIGHT

EXERCISE   SET   REPS   TEMPO   WEIGHT

EXERCISE   SET   REPS   TEMPO   WEIGHT

EXERCISE   SET   REPS   TEMPO   WEIGHT

EXERCISE   SET   REPS   TEMPO   WEIGHT

"Dear Body, I love you!

EXERCISE		SET	REPS	TEMPO	WEIGHT

EXERCISE		SET	REPS	TEMPO	WEIGHT

EXERCISE		SET	REPS	TEMPO	WEIGHT

EXERCISE		SET	REPS	TEMPO	WEIGHT

Notes

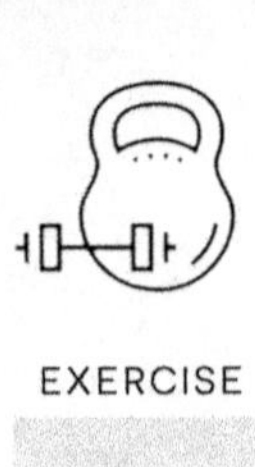

EXERCISE	SET	REPS	TEMPO	WEIGHT

EXERCISE	SET	REPS	TEMPO	WEIGHT

EXERCISE	SET	REPS	TEMPO	WEIGHT

EXERCISE	SET	REPS	TEMPO	WEIGHT

EXERCISE	SET	REPS	TEMPO	WEIGHT

EXERCISE	SET	REPS	TEMPO	WEIGHT

"Dear Body, I love you!

EXERCISE		SET	REPS	TEMPO	WEIGHT

EXERCISE		SET	REPS	TEMPO	WEIGHT

EXERCISE		SET	REPS	TEMPO	WEIGHT

EXERCISE		SET	REPS	TEMPO	WEIGHT

Notes

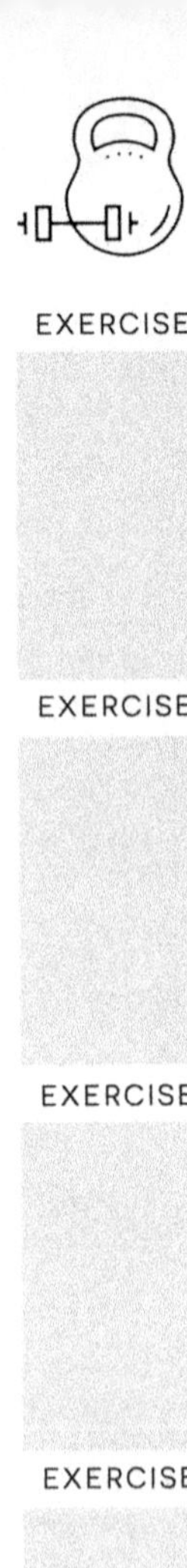

DATE: TIME:

MUSCLE GROUP:

EXERCISE	SET	REPS	TEMPO	WEIGHT

EXERCISE	SET	REPS	TEMPO	WEIGHT

EXERCISE	SET	REPS	TEMPO	WEIGHT

EXERCISE	SET	REPS	TEMPO	WEIGHT

EXERCISE	SET	REPS	TEMPO	WEIGHT

EXERCISE	SET	REPS	TEMPO	WEIGHT

"Dear Body, I love you!"

EXERCISE		SET	REPS	TEMPO	WEIGHT

EXERCISE		SET	REPS	TEMPO	WEIGHT

EXERCISE		SET	REPS	TEMPO	WEIGHT

EXERCISE		SET	REPS	TEMPO	WEIGHT

Notes

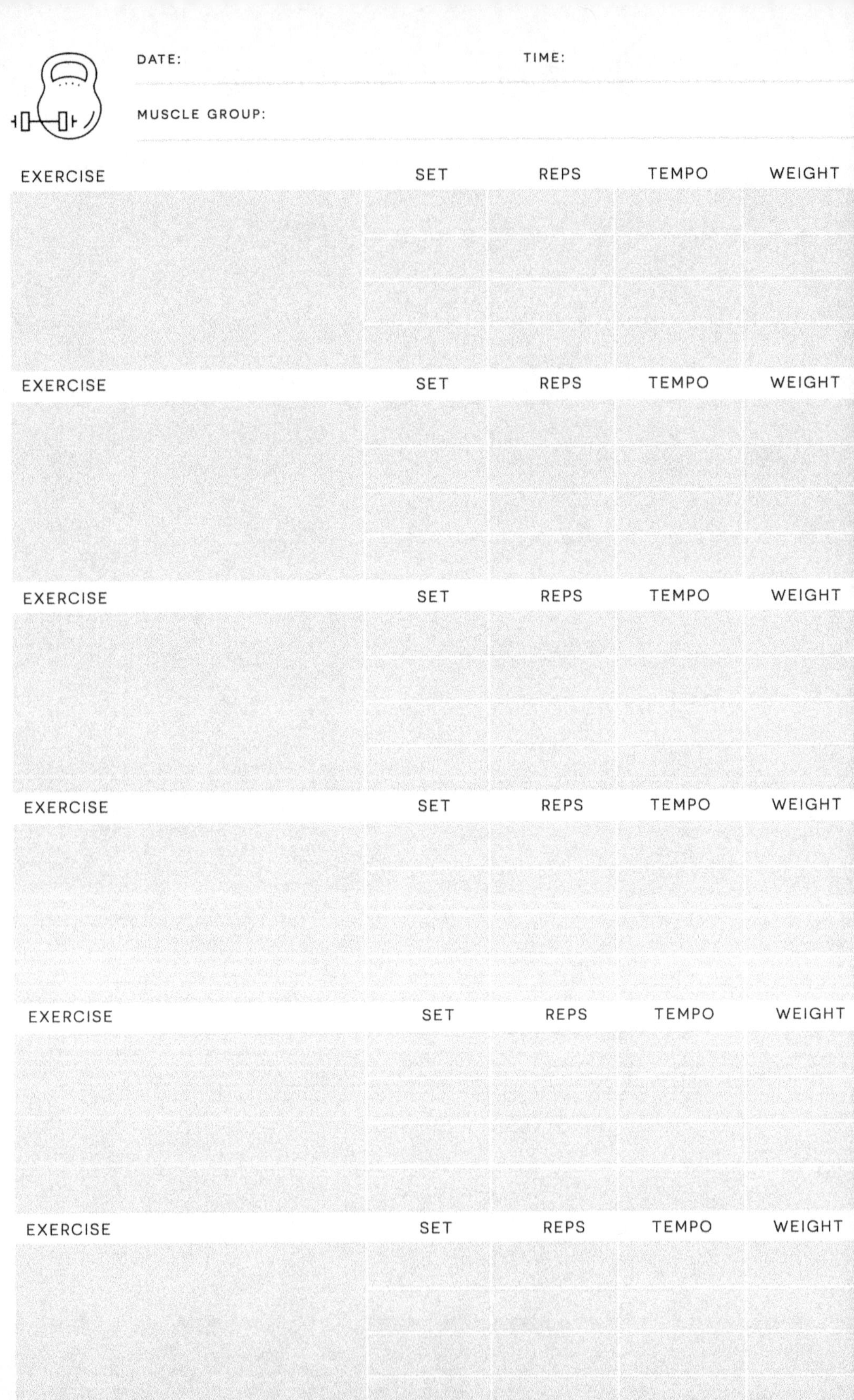

DATE:
TIME:
MUSCLE GROUP:
EXERCISE
SET
REPS
TEMPO
WEIGHT

"Dear Body, 1 love you!"

EXERCISE	SET	REPS	TEMPO	WEIGHT

EXERCISE	SET	REPS	TEMPO	WEIGHT

EXERCISE	SET	REPS	TEMPO	WEIGHT

EXERCISE	SET	REPS	TEMPO	WEIGHT

Notes

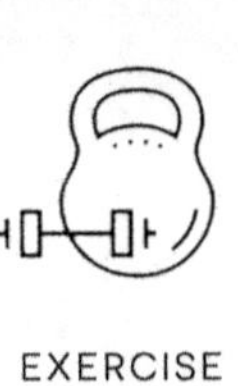

DATE:

TIME:

MUSCLE GROUP:

EXERCISE	SET	REPS	TEMPO	WEIGHT

EXERCISE	SET	REPS	TEMPO	WEIGHT

EXERCISE	SET	REPS	TEMPO	WEIGHT

EXERCISE	SET	REPS	TEMPO	WEIGHT

EXERCISE	SET	REPS	TEMPO	WEIGHT

EXERCISE	SET	REPS	TEMPO	WEIGHT

"Dear Body, I love you!

EXERCISE	SET	REPS	TEMPO	WEIGHT

EXERCISE	SET	REPS	TEMPO	WEIGHT

EXERCISE	SET	REPS	TEMPO	WEIGHT

EXERCISE	SET	REPS	TEMPO	WEIGHT

Notes

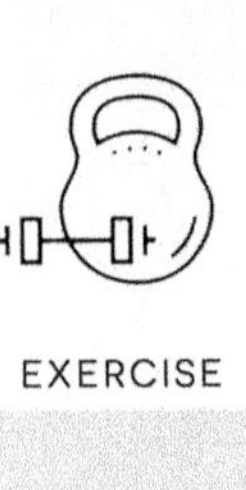

DATE:

TIME:

MUSCLE GROUP:

EXERCISE	SET	REPS	TEMPO	WEIGHT

EXERCISE	SET	REPS	TEMPO	WEIGHT

EXERCISE	SET	REPS	TEMPO	WEIGHT

EXERCISE	SET	REPS	TEMPO	WEIGHT

EXERCISE	SET	REPS	TEMPO	WEIGHT

EXERCISE	SET	REPS	TEMPO	WEIGHT

"Dear Body, I love you!

EXERCISE	SET	REPS	TEMPO	WEIGHT

EXERCISE	SET	REPS	TEMPO	WEIGHT

EXERCISE	SET	REPS	TEMPO	WEIGHT

EXERCISE	SET	REPS	TEMPO	WEIGHT

Notes

EXERCISE	SET	REPS	TEMPO	WEIGHT

EXERCISE	SET	REPS	TEMPO	WEIGHT

EXERCISE	SET	REPS	TEMPO	WEIGHT

EXERCISE	SET	REPS	TEMPO	WEIGHT

EXERCISE	SET	REPS	TEMPO	WEIGHT

EXERCISE	SET	REPS	TEMPO	WEIGHT

"Dear Body, 1 love you!"

EXERCISE		SET	REPS	TEMPO	WEIGHT

EXERCISE		SET	REPS	TEMPO	WEIGHT

EXERCISE		SET	REPS	TEMPO	WEIGHT

EXERCISE		SET	REPS	TEMPO	WEIGHT

Notes

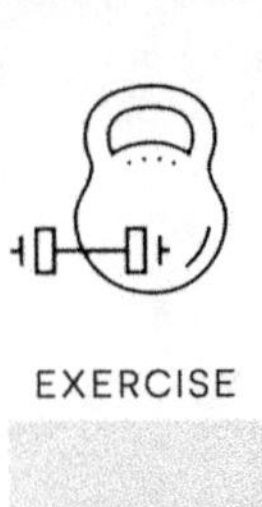

EXERCISE	SET	REPS	TEMPO	WEIGHT

EXERCISE	SET	REPS	TEMPO	WEIGHT

EXERCISE	SET	REPS	TEMPO	WEIGHT

EXERCISE	SET	REPS	TEMPO	WEIGHT

EXERCISE	SET	REPS	TEMPO	WEIGHT

EXERCISE	SET	REPS	TEMPO	WEIGHT

"Dear Body, I love you!"

EXERCISE	SET	REPS	TEMPO	WEIGHT

EXERCISE	SET	REPS	TEMPO	WEIGHT

EXERCISE	SET	REPS	TEMPO	WEIGHT

EXERCISE	SET	REPS	TEMPO	WEIGHT

Notes

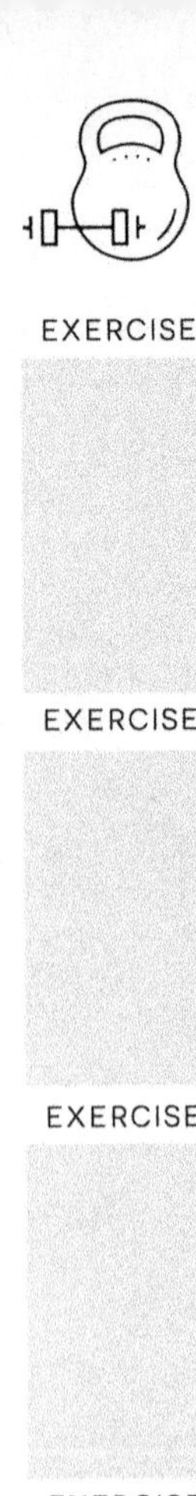

DATE: TIME:

MUSCLE GROUP:

EXERCISE	SET	REPS	TEMPO	WEIGHT

EXERCISE	SET	REPS	TEMPO	WEIGHT

EXERCISE	SET	REPS	TEMPO	WEIGHT

EXERCISE	SET	REPS	TEMPO	WEIGHT

EXERCISE	SET	REPS	TEMPO	WEIGHT

EXERCISE	SET	REPS	TEMPO	WEIGHT

EXERCISE	SET	REPS	TEMPO	WEIGHT

EXERCISE	SET	REPS	TEMPO	WEIGHT

EXERCISE	SET	REPS	TEMPO	WEIGHT

EXERCISE	SET	REPS	TEMPO	WEIGHT

Notes

EXERCISE	SET	REPS	TEMPO	WEIGHT

EXERCISE	SET	REPS	TEMPO	WEIGHT

EXERCISE	SET	REPS	TEMPO	WEIGHT

EXERCISE	SET	REPS	TEMPO	WEIGHT

EXERCISE	SET	REPS	TEMPO	WEIGHT

EXERCISE	SET	REPS	TEMPO	WEIGHT

EXERCISE		SET	REPS	TEMPO	WEIGHT

EXERCISE		SET	REPS	TEMPO	WEIGHT

EXERCISE		SET	REPS	TEMPO	WEIGHT

EXERCISE		SET	REPS	TEMPO	WEIGHT

Notes

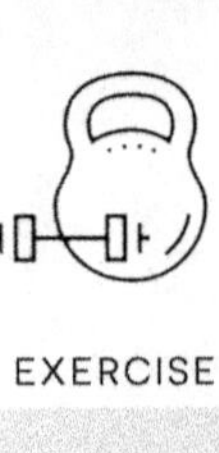

DATE:

TIME:

MUSCLE GROUP:

EXERCISE	SET	REPS	TEMPO	WEIGHT

EXERCISE	SET	REPS	TEMPO	WEIGHT

EXERCISE	SET	REPS	TEMPO	WEIGHT

EXERCISE	SET	REPS	TEMPO	WEIGHT

EXERCISE	SET	REPS	TEMPO	WEIGHT

EXERCISE	SET	REPS	TEMPO	WEIGHT

"Dear Body, I love you!

EXERCISE		SET	REPS	TEMPO	WEIGHT

EXERCISE		SET	REPS	TEMPO	WEIGHT

EXERCISE		SET	REPS	TEMPO	WEIGHT

EXERCISE		SET	REPS	TEMPO	WEIGHT

Notes

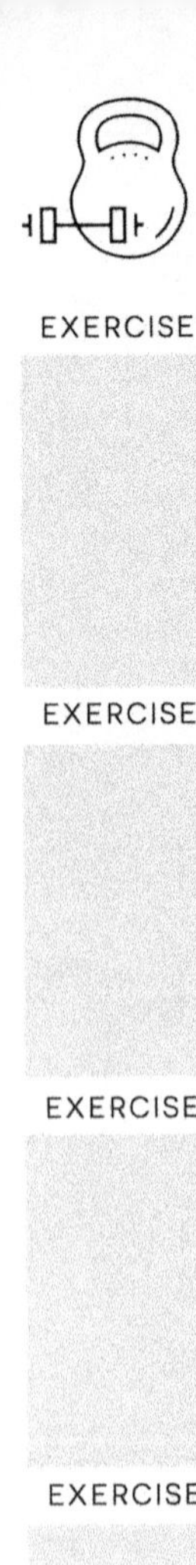

EXERCISE	SET	REPS	TEMPO	WEIGHT

EXERCISE	SET	REPS	TEMPO	WEIGHT

EXERCISE	SET	REPS	TEMPO	WEIGHT

EXERCISE	SET	REPS	TEMPO	WEIGHT

EXERCISE	SET	REPS	TEMPO	WEIGHT

EXERCISE	SET	REPS	TEMPO	WEIGHT

"Dear Body, I love you!"

EXERCISE	SET	REPS	TEMPO	WEIGHT

EXERCISE	SET	REPS	TEMPO	WEIGHT

EXERCISE	SET	REPS	TEMPO	WEIGHT

EXERCISE	SET	REPS	TEMPO	WEIGHT

Notes

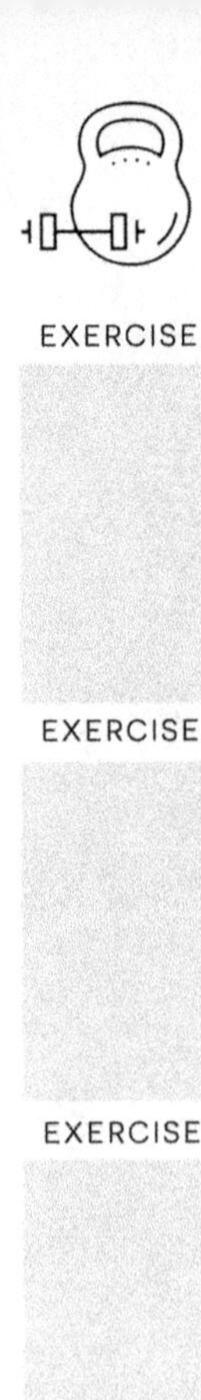

DATE: TIME:

MUSCLE GROUP:

EXERCISE	SET	REPS	TEMPO	WEIGHT

EXERCISE	SET	REPS	TEMPO	WEIGHT

EXERCISE	SET	REPS	TEMPO	WEIGHT

EXERCISE	SET	REPS	TEMPO	WEIGHT

EXERCISE	SET	REPS	TEMPO	WEIGHT

EXERCISE	SET	REPS	TEMPO	WEIGHT

EXERCISE		SET	REPS	TEMPO	WEIGHT

EXERCISE		SET	REPS	TEMPO	WEIGHT

EXERCISE		SET	REPS	TEMPO	WEIGHT

EXERCISE		SET	REPS	TEMPO	WEIGHT

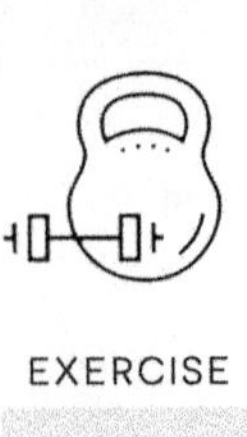

DATE: TIME:

MUSCLE GROUP:

EXERCISE	SET	REPS	TEMPO	WEIGHT

EXERCISE	SET	REPS	TEMPO	WEIGHT

EXERCISE	SET	REPS	TEMPO	WEIGHT

EXERCISE	SET	REPS	TEMPO	WEIGHT

EXERCISE	SET	REPS	TEMPO	WEIGHT

EXERCISE	SET	REPS	TEMPO	WEIGHT

"Dear Body, I love you!"

EXERCISE	SET	REPS	TEMPO	WEIGHT

EXERCISE	SET	REPS	TEMPO	WEIGHT

EXERCISE	SET	REPS	TEMPO	WEIGHT

EXERCISE	SET	REPS	TEMPO	WEIGHT

Notes

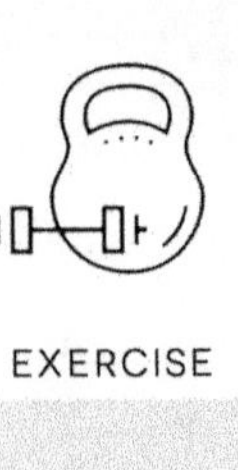

DATE:

TIME:

MUSCLE GROUP:

EXERCISE		SET	REPS	TEMPO	WEIGHT

EXERCISE		SET	REPS	TEMPO	WEIGHT

EXERCISE		SET	REPS	TEMPO	WEIGHT

EXERCISE		SET	REPS	TEMPO	WEIGHT

EXERCISE		SET	REPS	TEMPO	WEIGHT

EXERCISE		SET	REPS	TEMPO	WEIGHT

"Dear Body, I love you!"

EXERCISE	SET	REPS	TEMPO	WEIGHT

EXERCISE	SET	REPS	TEMPO	WEIGHT

EXERCISE	SET	REPS	TEMPO	WEIGHT

EXERCISE	SET	REPS	TEMPO	WEIGHT

Notes

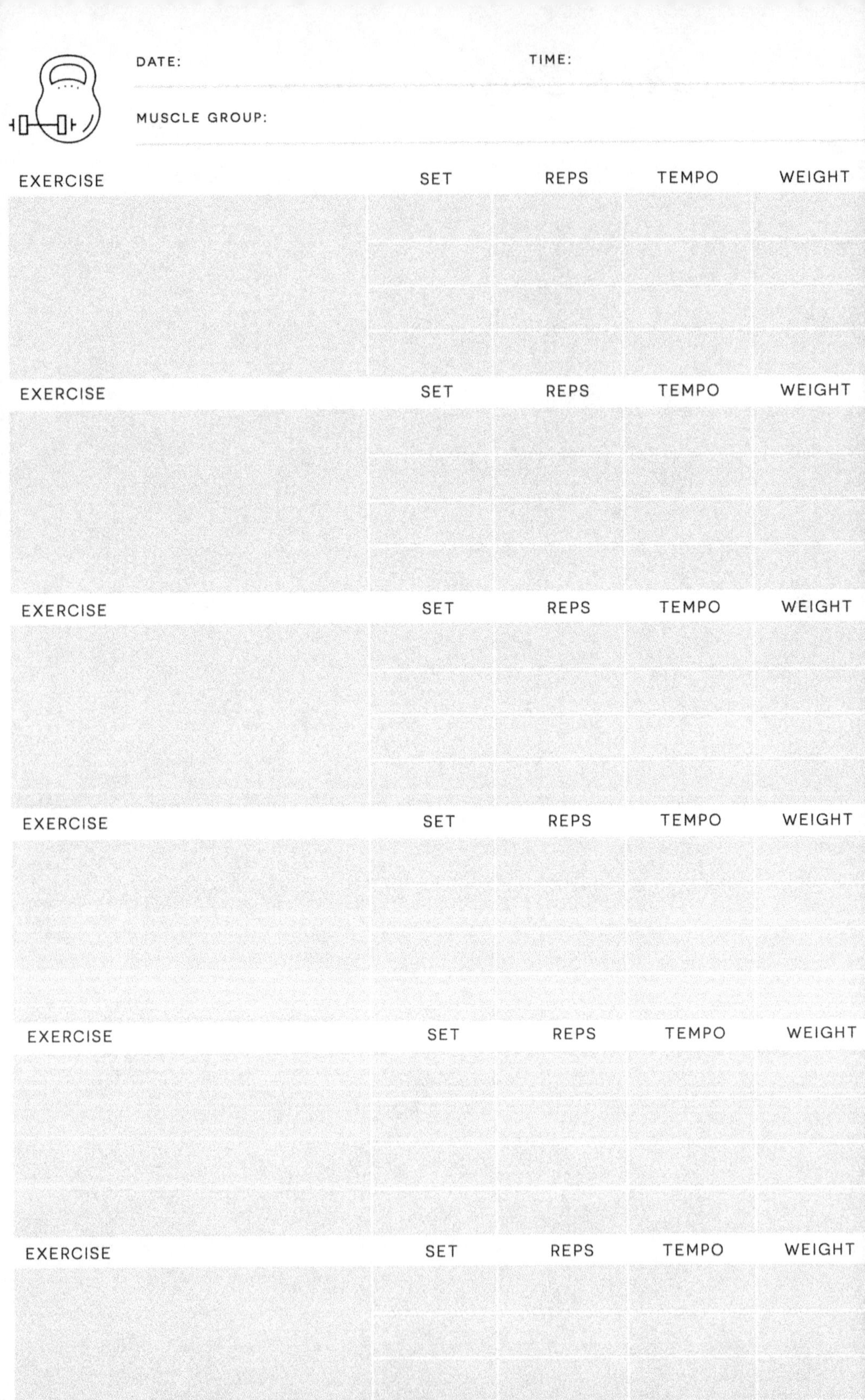

DATE:
TIME:
MUSCLE GROUP:
EXERCISE   SET   REPS   TEMPO   WEIGHT
EXERCISE   SET   REPS   TEMPO   WEIGHT
EXERCISE   SET   REPS   TEMPO   WEIGHT
EXERCISE   SET   REPS   TEMPO   WEIGHT
EXERCISE   SET   REPS   TEMPO   WEIGHT
EXERCISE   SET   REPS   TEMPO   WEIGHT

"Dear Body, I love you!"

EXERCISE				SET	REPS	TEMPO	WEIGHT

EXERCISE				SET	REPS	TEMPO	WEIGHT

EXERCISE				SET	REPS	TEMPO	WEIGHT

EXERCISE				SET	REPS	TEMPO	WEIGHT

Notes

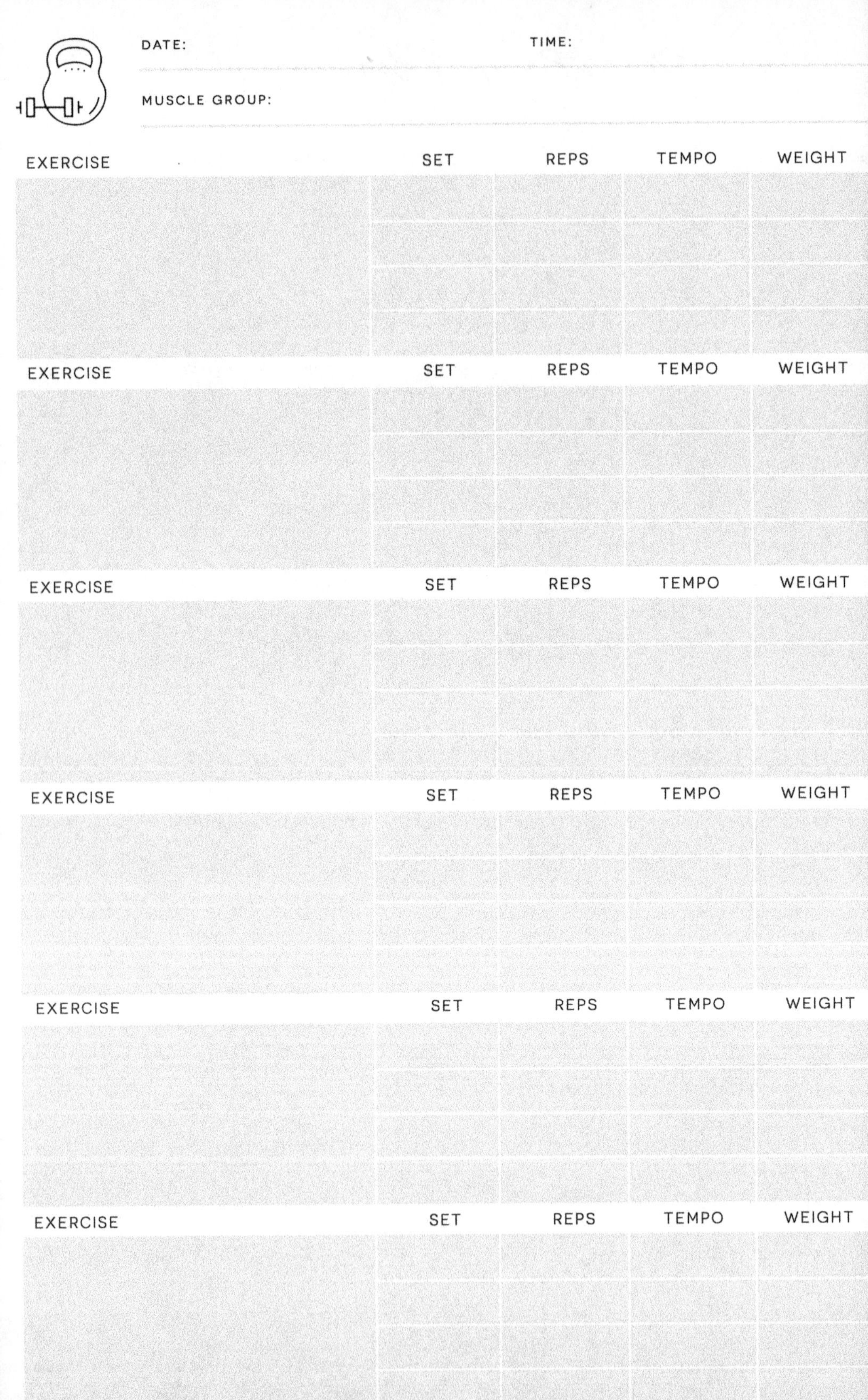

DATE:
TIME:
MUSCLE GROUP:

EXERCISE | SET | REPS | TEMPO | WEIGHT
EXERCISE | SET | REPS | TEMPO | WEIGHT
EXERCISE | SET | REPS | TEMPO | WEIGHT
EXERCISE | SET | REPS | TEMPO | WEIGHT
EXERCISE | SET | REPS | TEMPO | WEIGHT
EXERCISE | SET | REPS | TEMPO | WEIGHT

"Dear Body, I love you!"

EXERCISE	SET	REPS	TEMPO	WEIGHT

EXERCISE	SET	REPS	TEMPO	WEIGHT

EXERCISE	SET	REPS	TEMPO	WEIGHT

EXERCISE	SET	REPS	TEMPO	WEIGHT

Notes

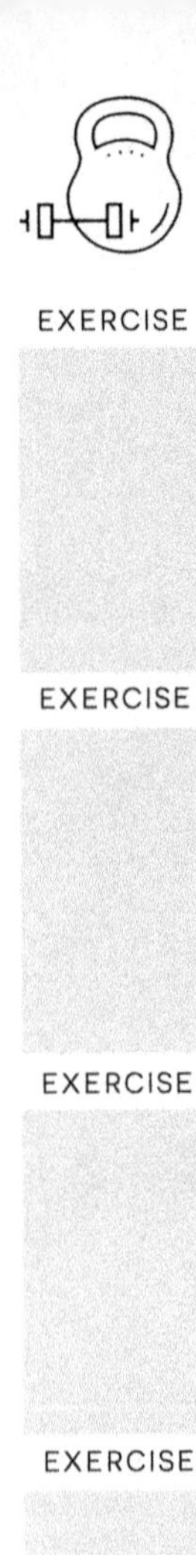

DATE:

TIME:

MUSCLE GROUP:

EXERCISE	SET	REPS	TEMPO	WEIGHT

EXERCISE	SET	REPS	TEMPO	WEIGHT

EXERCISE	SET	REPS	TEMPO	WEIGHT

EXERCISE	SET	REPS	TEMPO	WEIGHT

EXERCISE	SET	REPS	TEMPO	WEIGHT

EXERCISE	SET	REPS	TEMPO	WEIGHT

"Dear Body, I love you!"

EXERCISE	SET	REPS	TEMPO	WEIGHT

EXERCISE	SET	REPS	TEMPO	WEIGHT

EXERCISE	SET	REPS	TEMPO	WEIGHT

EXERCISE	SET	REPS	TEMPO	WEIGHT

Notes

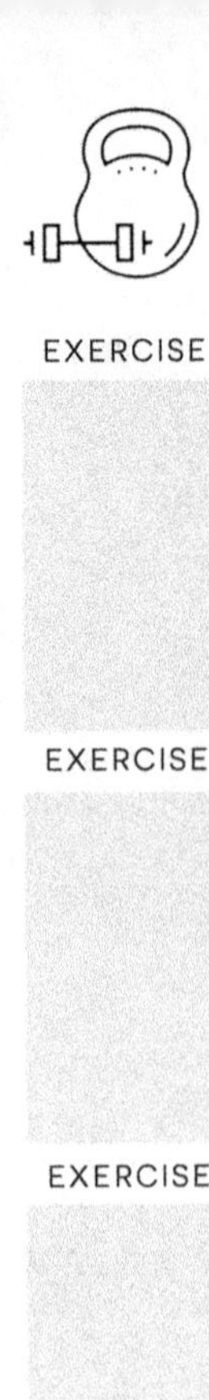

EXERCISE	SET	REPS	TEMPO	WEIGHT

EXERCISE	SET	REPS	TEMPO	WEIGHT

EXERCISE	SET	REPS	TEMPO	WEIGHT

EXERCISE	SET	REPS	TEMPO	WEIGHT

EXERCISE	SET	REPS	TEMPO	WEIGHT

EXERCISE	SET	REPS	TEMPO	WEIGHT

"Dear Body, I love you!"

EXERCISE	SET	REPS	TEMPO	WEIGHT

EXERCISE	SET	REPS	TEMPO	WEIGHT

EXERCISE	SET	REPS	TEMPO	WEIGHT

EXERCISE	SET	REPS	TEMPO	WEIGHT

Notes

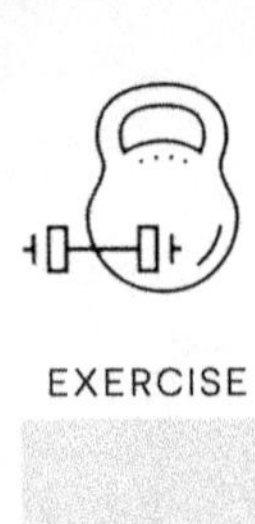

EXERCISE	SET	REPS	TEMPO	WEIGHT

EXERCISE	SET	REPS	TEMPO	WEIGHT

EXERCISE	SET	REPS	TEMPO	WEIGHT

EXERCISE	SET	REPS	TEMPO	WEIGHT

EXERCISE	SET	REPS	TEMPO	WEIGHT

EXERCISE	SET	REPS	TEMPO	WEIGHT

"Dear Body, I love you!"

EXERCISE		SET	REPS	TEMPO	WEIGHT

EXERCISE		SET	REPS	TEMPO	WEIGHT

EXERCISE		SET	REPS	TEMPO	WEIGHT

EXERCISE		SET	REPS	TEMPO	WEIGHT

Notes

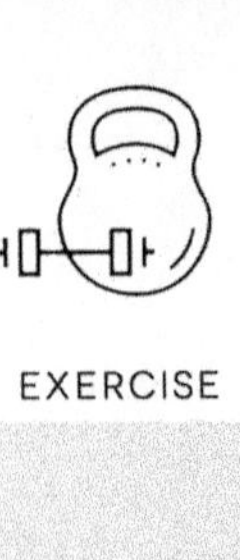

DATE: TIME:

MUSCLE GROUP:

EXERCISE	SET	REPS	TEMPO	WEIGHT

EXERCISE	SET	REPS	TEMPO	WEIGHT

EXERCISE	SET	REPS	TEMPO	WEIGHT

EXERCISE	SET	REPS	TEMPO	WEIGHT

EXERCISE	SET	REPS	TEMPO	WEIGHT

EXERCISE	SET	REPS	TEMPO	WEIGHT

EXERCISE	SET	REPS	TEMPO	WEIGHT

EXERCISE	SET	REPS	TEMPO	WEIGHT

EXERCISE	SET	REPS	TEMPO	WEIGHT

EXERCISE	SET	REPS	TEMPO	WEIGHT

Notes

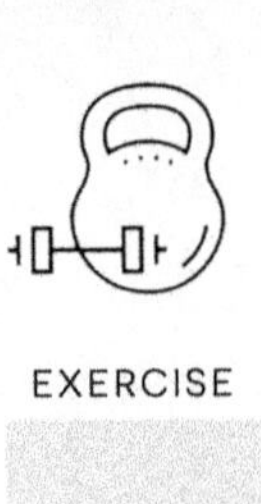

EXERCISE	SET	REPS	TEMPO	WEIGHT

EXERCISE	SET	REPS	TEMPO	WEIGHT

EXERCISE	SET	REPS	TEMPO	WEIGHT

EXERCISE	SET	REPS	TEMPO	WEIGHT

EXERCISE	SET	REPS	TEMPO	WEIGHT

EXERCISE	SET	REPS	TEMPO	WEIGHT

EXERCISE | SET | REPS | TEMPO | WEIGHT

EXERCISE | SET | REPS | TEMPO | WEIGHT

EXERCISE | SET | REPS | TEMPO | WEIGHT

EXERCISE | SET | REPS | TEMPO | WEIGHT

Notes

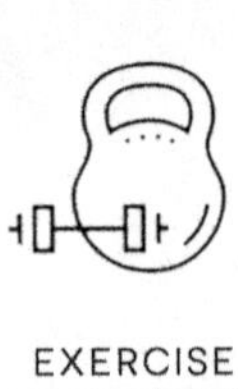

DATE: TIME:

MUSCLE GROUP:

EXERCISE	SET	REPS	TEMPO	WEIGHT

EXERCISE	SET	REPS	TEMPO	WEIGHT

EXERCISE	SET	REPS	TEMPO	WEIGHT

EXERCISE	SET	REPS	TEMPO	WEIGHT

EXERCISE	SET	REPS	TEMPO	WEIGHT

EXERCISE	SET	REPS	TEMPO	WEIGHT

"Dear Body, I love you!"

EXERCISE	SET	REPS	TEMPO	WEIGHT

EXERCISE	SET	REPS	TEMPO	WEIGHT

EXERCISE	SET	REPS	TEMPO	WEIGHT

EXERCISE	SET	REPS	TEMPO	WEIGHT

Notes

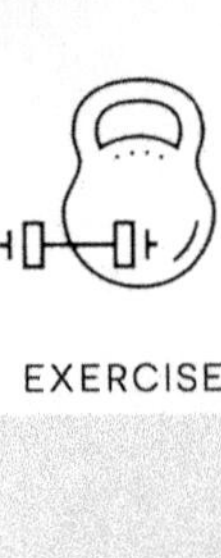

EXERCISE	SET	REPS	TEMPO	WEIGHT

EXERCISE	SET	REPS	TEMPO	WEIGHT

EXERCISE	SET	REPS	TEMPO	WEIGHT

EXERCISE	SET	REPS	TEMPO	WEIGHT

EXERCISE	SET	REPS	TEMPO	WEIGHT

EXERCISE	SET	REPS	TEMPO	WEIGHT

"Dear Body, I love you!"

EXERCISE		SET	REPS	TEMPO	WEIGHT

EXERCISE		SET	REPS	TEMPO	WEIGHT

EXERCISE		SET	REPS	TEMPO	WEIGHT

EXERCISE		SET	REPS	TEMPO	WEIGHT

Notes

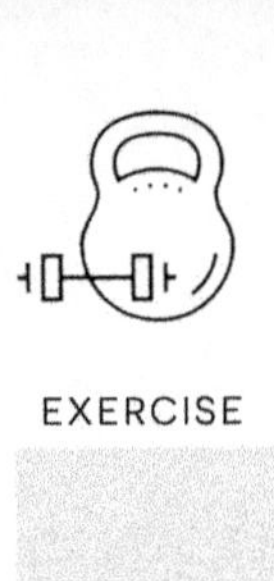

DATE:

TIME:

MUSCLE GROUP:

EXERCISE		SET	REPS	TEMPO	WEIGHT

EXERCISE		SET	REPS	TEMPO	WEIGHT

EXERCISE		SET	REPS	TEMPO	WEIGHT

EXERCISE		SET	REPS	TEMPO	WEIGHT

EXERCISE		SET	REPS	TEMPO	WEIGHT

EXERCISE		SET	REPS	TEMPO	WEIGHT

"Dear Body, I love you!"

EXERCISE	SET	REPS	TEMPO	WEIGHT

EXERCISE	SET	REPS	TEMPO	WEIGHT

EXERCISE	SET	REPS	TEMPO	WEIGHT

EXERCISE	SET	REPS	TEMPO	WEIGHT

Notes

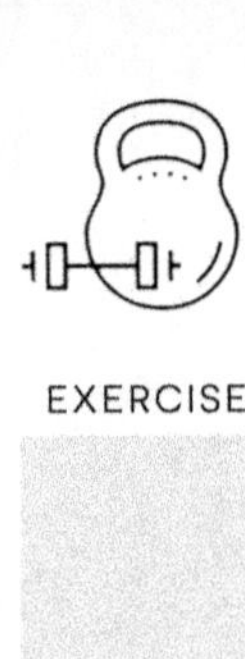

EXERCISE	SET	REPS	TEMPO	WEIGHT

EXERCISE	SET	REPS	TEMPO	WEIGHT

EXERCISE	SET	REPS	TEMPO	WEIGHT

EXERCISE	SET	REPS	TEMPO	WEIGHT

EXERCISE	SET	REPS	TEMPO	WEIGHT

EXERCISE	SET	REPS	TEMPO	WEIGHT

"Dear Body, I love you!"

EXERCISE		SET	REPS	TEMPO	WEIGHT

EXERCISE		SET	REPS	TEMPO	WEIGHT

EXERCISE		SET	REPS	TEMPO	WEIGHT

EXERCISE		SET	REPS	TEMPO	WEIGHT

Notes

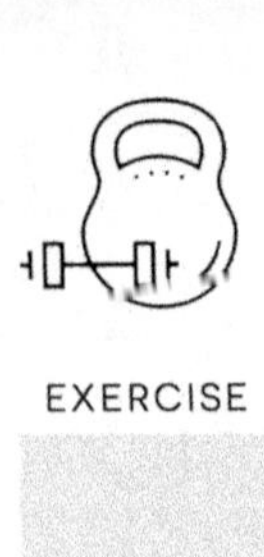

DATE: TIME:

MUSCLE GROUP:

EXERCISE	SET	REPS	TEMPO	WEIGHT

EXERCISE	SET	REPS	TEMPO	WEIGHT

EXERCISE	SET	REPS	TEMPO	WEIGHT

EXERCISE	SET	REPS	TEMPO	WEIGHT

EXERCISE	SET	REPS	TEMPO	WEIGHT

EXERCISE	SET	REPS	TEMPO	WEIGHT

"Dear Body, I love you!"

EXERCISE	SET	REPS	TEMPO	WEIGHT

EXERCISE	SET	REPS	TEMPO	WEIGHT

EXERCISE	SET	REPS	TEMPO	WEIGHT

EXERCISE	SET	REPS	TEMPO	WEIGHT

Notes

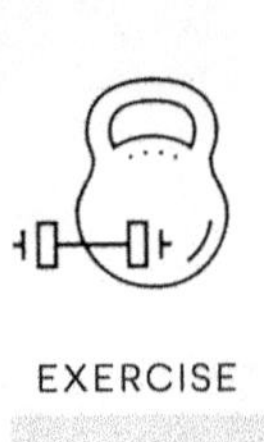

EXERCISE	SET	REPS	TEMPO	WEIGHT

EXERCISE	SET	REPS	TEMPO	WEIGHT

EXERCISE	SET	REPS	TEMPO	WEIGHT

EXERCISE	SET	REPS	TEMPO	WEIGHT

EXERCISE	SET	REPS	TEMPO	WEIGHT

EXERCISE	SET	REPS	TEMPO	WEIGHT

"Dear Body, I love you!

EXERCISE		SET	REPS	TEMPO	WEIGHT

EXERCISE		SET	REPS	TEMPO	WEIGHT

EXERCISE		SET	REPS	TEMPO	WEIGHT

EXERCISE		SET	REPS	TEMPO	WEIGHT

Notes

Smashed it